THE STRANGER

I CALL

GRANDMA

Swanee Ballman

illustrated by

Stephanie Brunson

Jawbone Publishing Corporation St. Cloud, FL

www.jawbonepublishing.com

Published by Jawbone Publishing Corporation
3875 Crosley Avenue
Saint Cloud, FL 34772-8150

Printed in Hong Kong

Library of Congress Control Number: 2001126200

ISBN: 0-9702959-4-4

CHAPTER ONE

I have some really neat memories of
my grandfather.
He always hugged me and did lots of
things with ME!

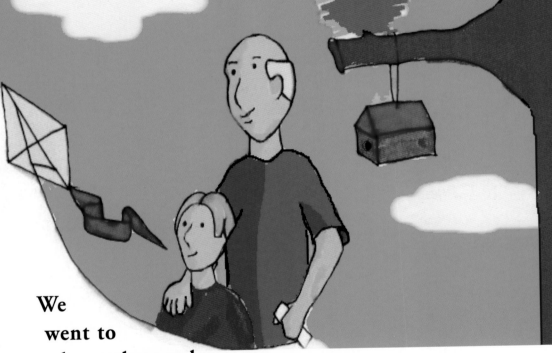

We
went to
the park together
and played ball. We watched TV together.
He even let me mess around with all the
tools in his garage.
He helped me build a birdhouse, and he
made an aluminum foil kite for me.

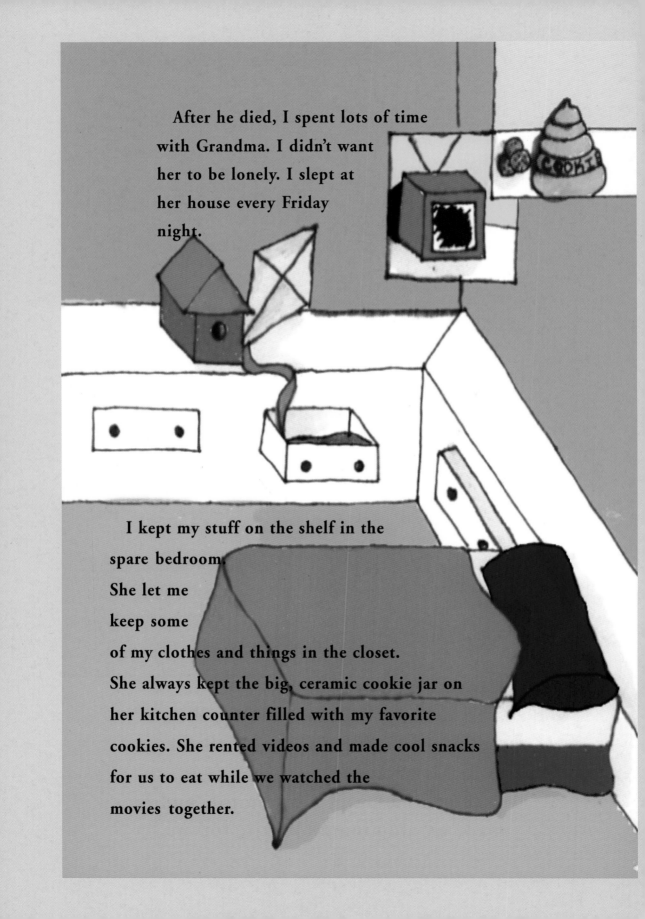

After he died, I spent lots of time with Grandma. I didn't want her to be lonely. I slept at her house every Friday night.

I kept my stuff on the shelf in the spare bedroom. She let me keep some of my clothes and things in the closet. She always kept the big, ceramic cookie jar on her kitchen counter filled with my favorite cookies. She rented videos and made cool snacks for us to eat while we watched the movies together.

One morning before school, while I
ate my breakfast, the telephone rang.
Dad answered it. I knew something was
wrong when he kept repeating the same words
to Grandma. He frowned and shook his
head as he talked.

When he hung up, he said
to my mom, "She's gone
off the deep end."

"What does that mean?"
I asked.

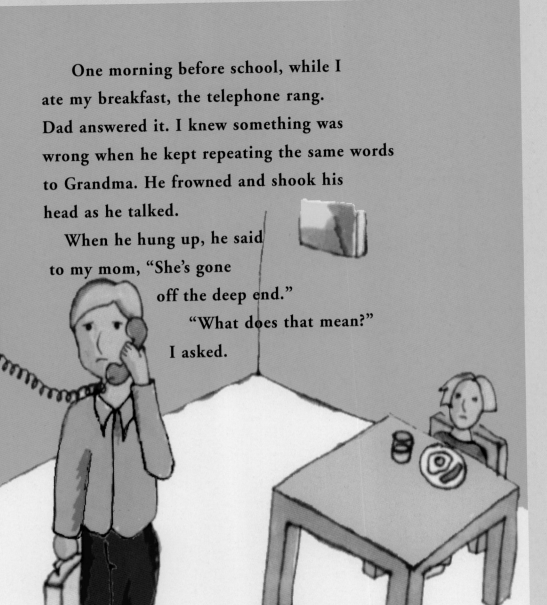

Andy," Mom said, "Grandma has a disease.
You know how she worries about little things ...
like they're major deals. And you've noticed how
she never wants to go anywhere anymore."

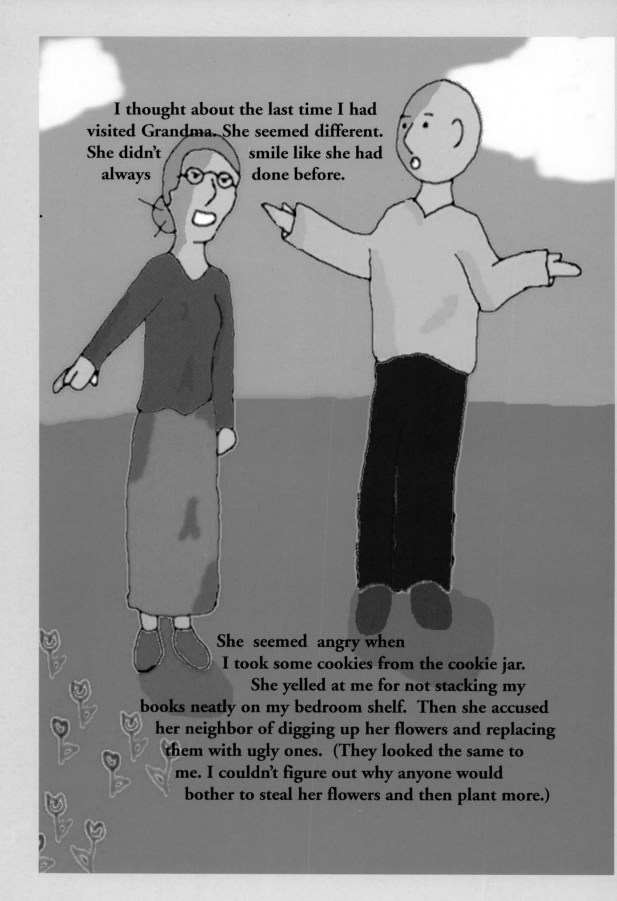

I thought about the last time I had visited Grandma. She seemed different. She didn't always smile like she had done before.

She seemed angry when I took some cookies from the cookie jar. She yelled at me for not stacking my books neatly on my bedroom shelf. Then she accused her neighbor of digging up her flowers and replacing them with ugly ones. (They looked the same to me. I couldn't figure out why anyone would bother to steal her flowers and then plant more.)

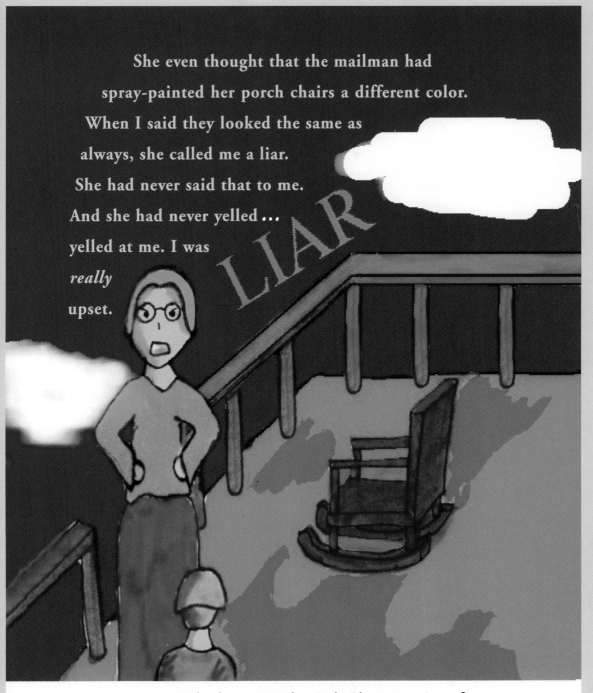

She even thought that the mailman had
spray-painted her porch chairs a different color.
When I said they looked the same as
always, she called me a liar.
She had never said that to me.
And she had never yelled...
yelled at me. I was
really
upset.

LIAR

I ran to my bedroom and cried. She came in a few
minutes later and said she was sorry. We
hugged. I figured she just had a bad
day. I have those sometimes, too.

Dad interrupted my thoughts. He leaned over and patted my hand. "Andy, Grandma can't take care of herself anymore."

To me, Grandma looked the same. She didn't look sick.

But I thought about the strange way she had been acting. She didn't call any of her friends anymore. She sat in her house with the drapes closed, and she always wore the same dress. Most of all, she didn't seem to care about me. She never asked me about school, or my friends, or anything.

"Andy," Dad said, "Grandma is going to move in with us. She will live here now."

Wow! That scared me. Grandma must *really* be sick.

"Will she get better?" I asked. "Will she go back home some day?"

"Probably not," Mom said. "She may get worse. She needs us to love and care for her."

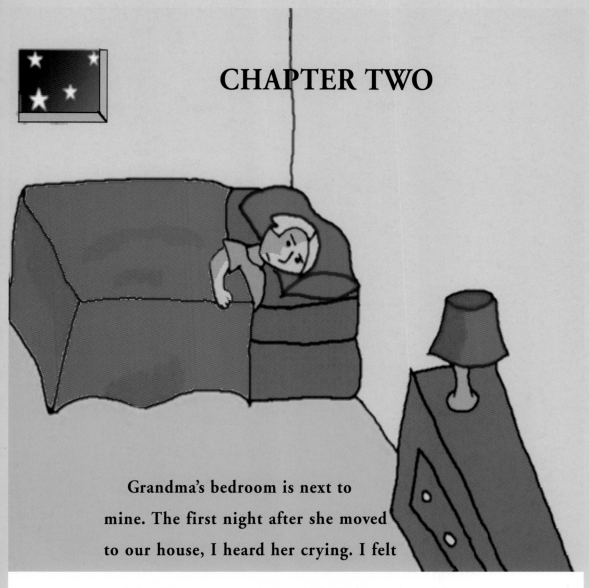

CHAPTER TWO

Grandma's bedroom is next to mine. The first night after she moved to our house, I heard her crying. I felt sad for her. I wanted to tell her that I loved her, but I just couldn't right then. I was still upset because she had screamed at me during dinner.

All night long, Grandma walked up and down the hall. She slammed her door many times. I couldn't sleep. My parents didn't sleep, either.

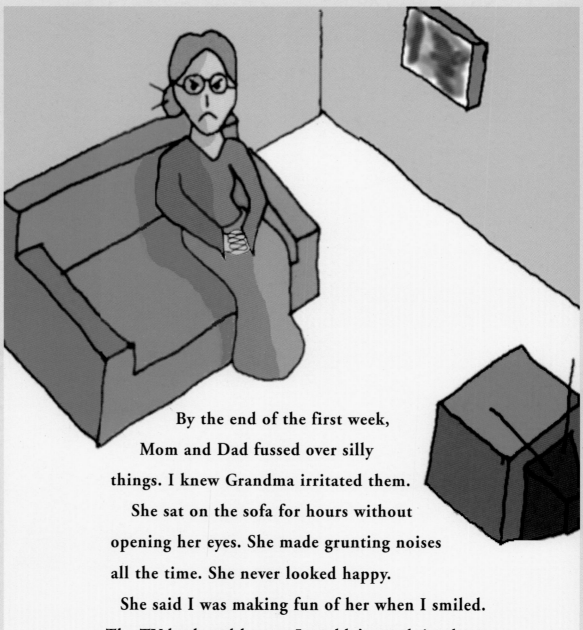

By the end of the first week,
Mom and Dad fussed over silly
things. I knew Grandma irritated them.
    She sat on the sofa for hours without
opening her eyes. She made grunting noises
all the time. She never looked happy.
    She said I was making fun of her when I smiled.
The TV bothered her, so I couldn't watch it whenever
she sat on the sofa. It seemed like she *always* sat
on the sofa.
    According to Grandma, everything I did was
wrong. She wasn't any fun to be around anymore.

Every dinner, she complained about living with us.
She told Mom and Dad that they were stealing her
money. After dinner, she went to
her bedroom Then, after we went
to bed, she came out and sat on the
sofa in the dark. I could hear her

grunting and talking to herself.
She did this every
night.

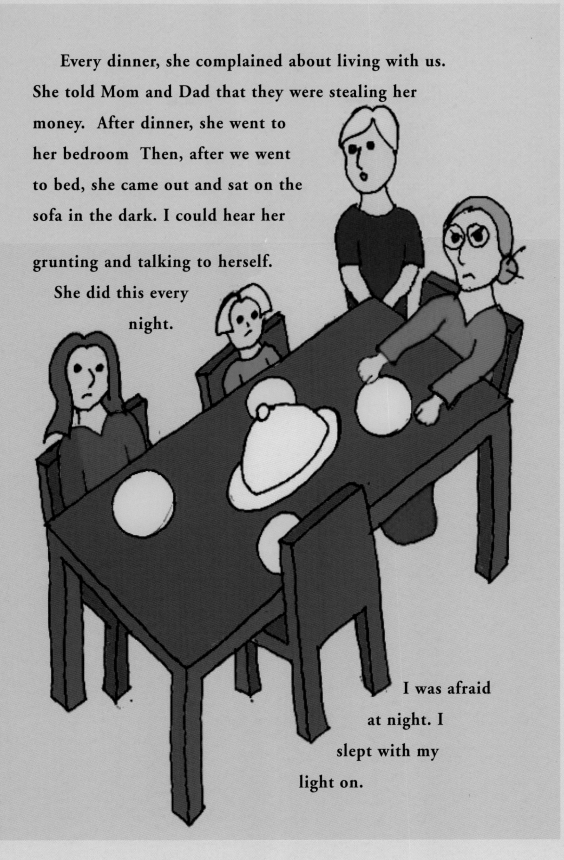

I was afraid
at night. I
slept with my
light on.

Almost every night she banged on my parent's bedroom door.

"I'm in big trouble," she'd shout. "The police are going to arrest me!" Or she'd yell, "Call the bank right now. I need to 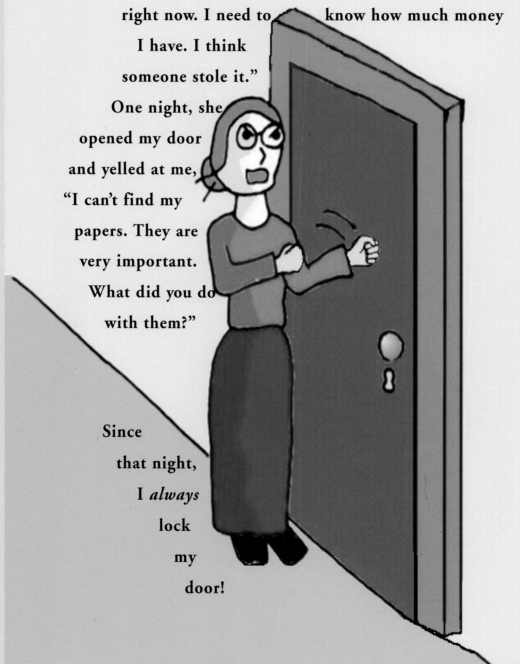 know how much money I have. I think someone stole it."

One night, she opened my door and yelled at me, "I can't find my papers. They are very important. What did you do with them?"

Since that night, I *always* lock my door!

Grandma had messed up my life
BIG time. My friends couldn't come to
my house after school anymore, because
Grandma couldn't stand any noise.

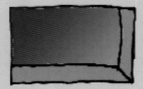

Mom couldn't drive me places, because
Grandma refused to go out of
the house. We couldn't leave her alone.

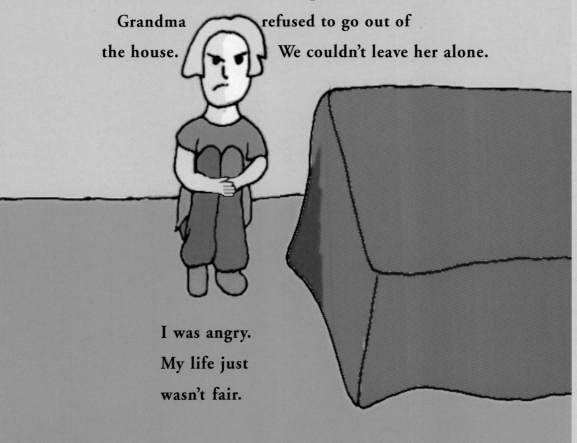

I was angry.
My life just
wasn't fair.

One afternoon, Grandma's eyes

grew big and dark. They looked like

someone had sprayed a coat of shiny

varnish on them. She looked very, very

mean.

She scared me.
I ran into
my bedroom
and slammed
the door.
I never wanted
to see Grandma
again.

Mom came into my room and sat on
the bed beside me.

"I know that life isn't good for you now,
honey," she said. "I'm so sorry. But
Grandma needs us. She's very sick."

"She's not sick!" I shouted. "She's just ...
just mean. I hate her!"

I cried and cried. "She doesn't want us to
be happy. I can't laugh, because that
bothers her. My friends can't come over to
play. I can't even watch
TV. And I can't
sleep at night.

I'm scared
of her. Why
can't she go back
to her house and be miserable all by herself?"

"This is her home now, Andy," Mom said. "Grandma can't take a pill and get well. We can't let her go back to her house, because she might hurt herself."

I wanted to scream, but I didn't. I knew Mom was trying very hard to help. She had dark circles under her eyes from not sleeping at night.

"You keep saying she's sick, Mom," I said. "I don't think she's sick. I think she just wants us to be as miserable as she is."

Mom sighed. "Yes, she is quite sick. You can't tell, because her sickness is in her brain. Each day, a little more of her memory dies. She doesn't know that she's acting mean. Someday, she won't know who we are."

I groaned. "I feel like I"m a bad kid, but I haven't done anything wrong. My friends don't think Grandma is sick.

They think she's weird and you're mean for not letting them come over here any more. They don't want me to come to

their houses now."

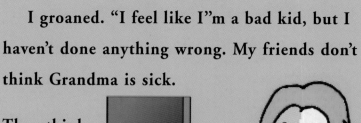

Mom nodded. "I know, honey," she said. "Tell then Grandma has Alzheimer's Disease. Have them ask their parents about it. That should help."

"What's it called ... Alls hammers?" I asked.

Mom laughed. It was great to see her smile. "It does sound like that!" she said. The man who discovered this disease was a Dr. Alzheimer."

Suddenly, I was scared. "Will Grandma die from Alz ... this disease?"

Mom didn't answer me right away. I think she was about to cry.

"Yes," she finally said. "Eventually, she will. How long that will be, we don't know. Her brain is slowly shutting down. When her brain no longer sends messages to the rest of her body - like to her heart and her lungs - she will die. Or, she may develop another illness that she

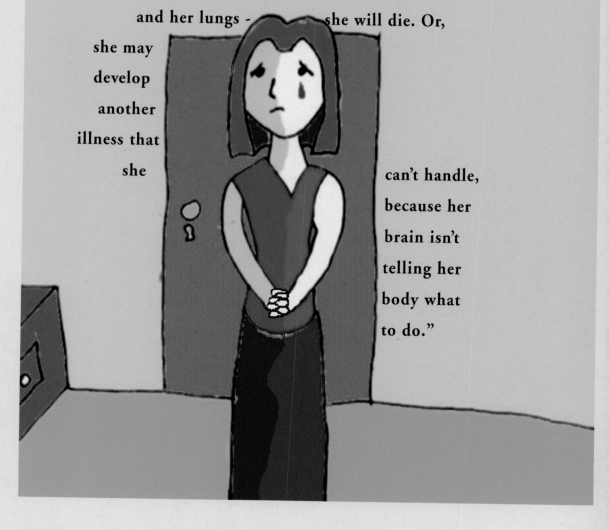

can't handle, because her brain isn't telling her body what to do."

Mom walked over to my desk, where I had been working on a jigsaw puzzle.

"Your puzzle is missing lots of pieces right now," she said. "Oh, they're here. But until you find the right place to put them into the pattern, you will have blank spots in your puzzle."

She pointed to the half-finished picture. "What happens if you misplace lots of pieces?"

I walked over to my desk and looked down at the puzzle.

"That's easy," I said. "I couldn't finish the puzzle."

Mom ruffled my hair. "Such a smart kid! Would you be upset if you lost pieces?"

"Sure, I would! I want to see the whole picture," I told her.

Mom picked up some pieces and dropped them into my hand. Grandma's brain is like this," she said. "Some pieces are lost and will never be found. Other pieces are there, but she can't fit them into the picture without first finding the missing pieces. Each day, more pieces disappear."

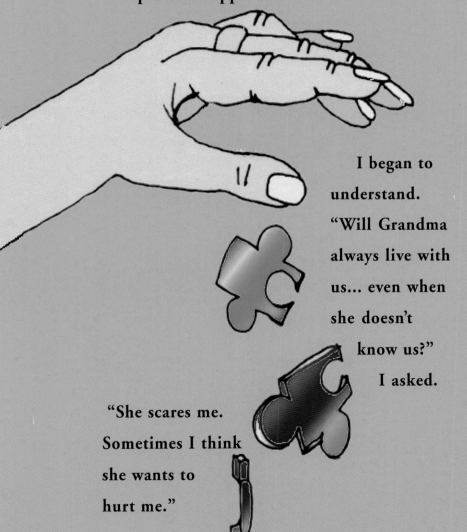

I began to understand. "Will Grandma always live with us... even when she doesn't know us?" I asked.

"She scares me. Sometimes I think she wants to hurt me."

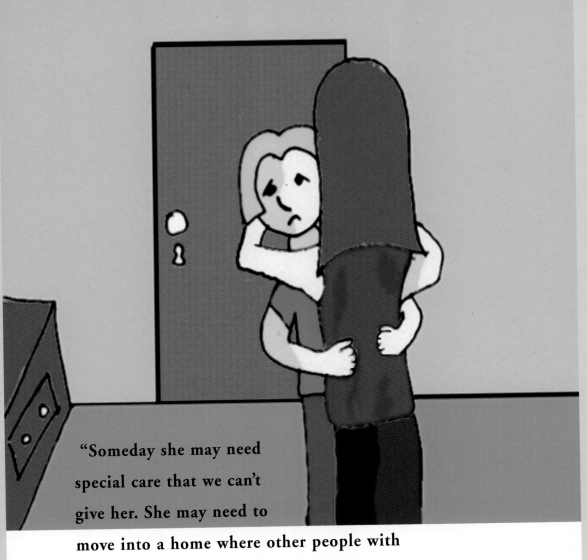

"Someday she may need special care that we can't give her. She may need to move into a home where other people with Alzheimer's live. Nurses trained to deal with people like Grandma work there. But for now, she needs us."

I dropped the puzzle pieces onto the desk. "I still don't like her." I felt bad that I said that.

Mom kissed me. "It's not Grandma that you dislike. You hate the disease that stole her mind."

Suddenly I had a scary thought.
What if my parents got Alzheimer's,
too? Maybe it's contagious. Then, I
would be all alone. Or I could get it, too.
"Will you and Dad get Alz ...
Alzheimer's? Will I get it?"

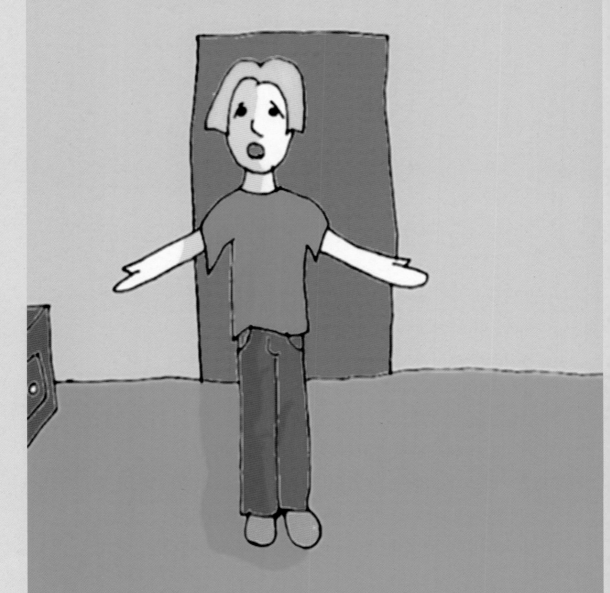

Mom shook her head. "Alzheimer's isn't contagious, like measles or chicken pox. And I can't promise that years from now, your dad or I won't get it. But, I can tell you this. Grandma is the only one in our family to have ever gotten this disease."

That made me feel better.

"She makes you and Dad mad, too, doesn't she?" I asked.

Mom nodded. "I sometimes forget that she's so sick. She doesn't realize that she screams such horrible things at us. I shouldn't snap at her, but sometimes I just can't help myself. Just like you, Andy, I'm trying hard to understand her. And, yes, it's tough being patient with someone who doesn't seem to appreciate what I do for her."

I looked at my mom's eyes. They were
filled with tears. "She makes you cry lots,
doesn't she?" I asked.

Mom sniffled. She blinked and tears
glistened in her eyelashes. I knew she was
pretending to be happy for me.

"If Grandma's brain were healthy,"
she said, "she would never, ever,
do the things she does.
And she would
never have
screamed at any
of us. You
know
that."

I love my mother. I didn't want her to be sad.
"I used to love Grandma. Now I don't," I said.

"Think of how she loved you before she got
sick," she said. "Think of all the wonderful times
you had together. That was your grandma."

That was tough for me to do. I could only think
of the way Grandma was acting now.
"Why should I love her
when she doesn't love me?"

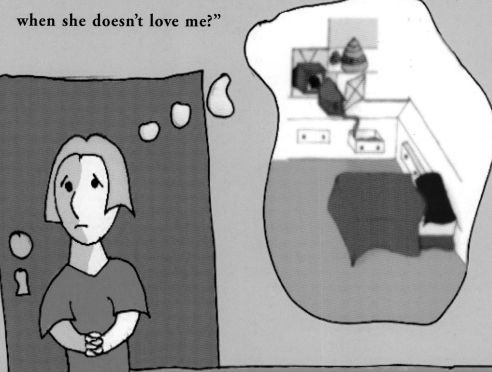

"The grandma who's trapped inside still loves you.
She's still the same grandmother who bought
cookies and watched TV with you," Mom said.

I knew what Mom was telling me, but I had trouble remembering the way Grandma once was.

"She isn't Grandma anymore. She won't ever be Grandma again," I said. "She's nothing like my Grandma. She's a stranger who's ruining my life. I want her to go away today."

Mom still didn't get angry. She just nodded. "Andy, she may not be living with us much longer. While she still knows us, we want to care for her. When you were little and needed for her to love you - even when you were naughty - Grandma always stood up for you. She loved you through temper-fits, even through coloring her pretty wallpaper with red crayon.

Now it's time to love her, no matter what."

Just then, Grandma knocked on my bedroom door.

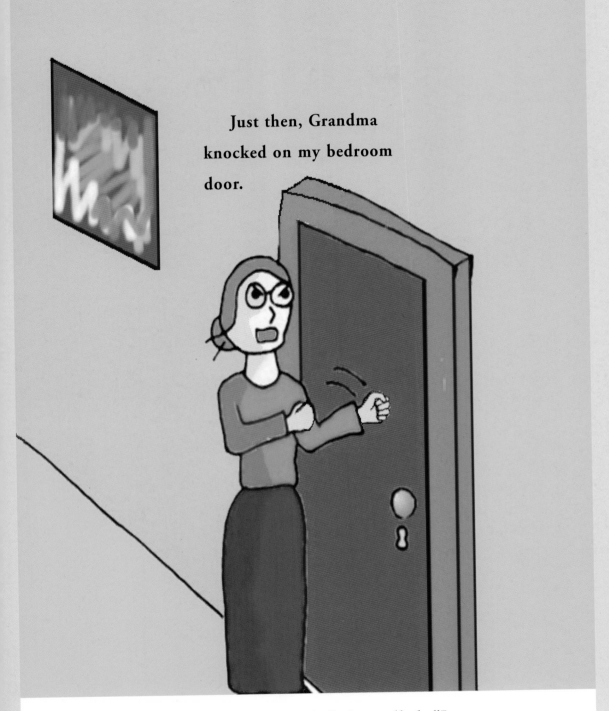

"I know you're in there, Andy," she yelled. "I
can't find my purse. I know you took it. I want it back."

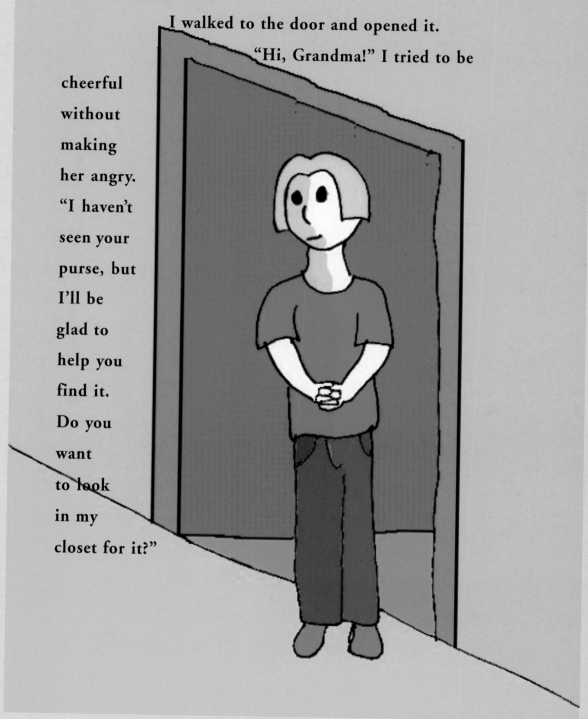

Mom winked at me. "Give it to her, kid!" she teased.

I walked to the door and opened it. "Hi, Grandma!" I tried to be cheerful without making her angry. "I haven't seen your purse, but I'll be glad to help you find it. Do you want to look in my closet for it?"

I took her hand and led her to the closet
door. She squinted her eyes and made her
funny little grunting noises.

As she leaned over to look at the closet
floor, she mumbled something. I didn't hear
what she said, but I knew she was complaining.

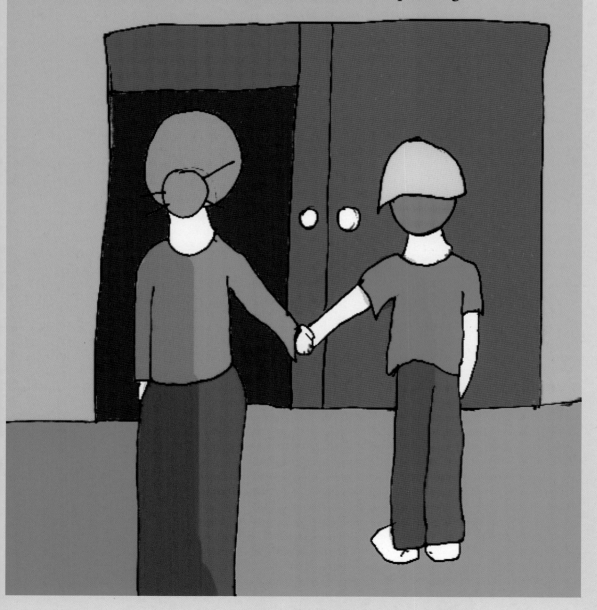

Mom patted my back. "You know, Andy, that's a terrific idea! We'll all work together to solve this problem."

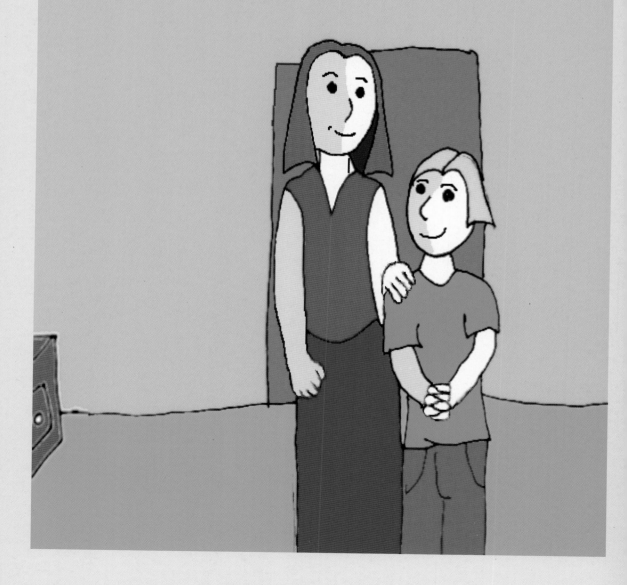

I turned to smile at my mother.
She smiled back at me. Smiling made
me feel good.

"Okay, Mom. I think I can do that."
Mom winked. "I'm sure you can,
honey. I'm sure you can!"

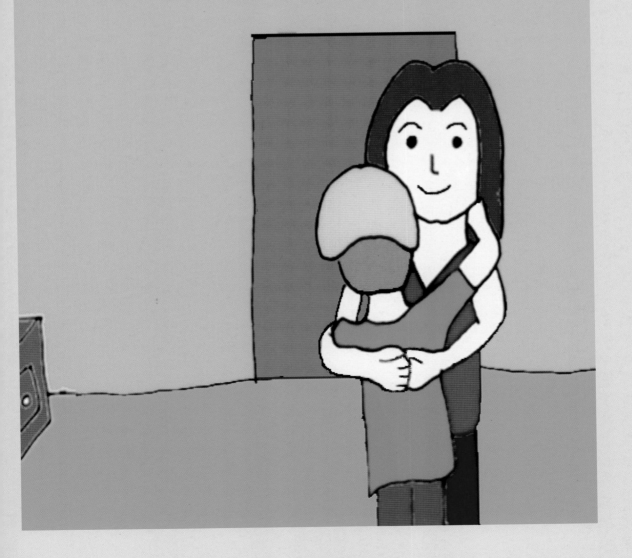

All forms of dementia are heartbreaking, for the one suffering from this debilitating mental illness and for those who care for the patient.

So often the characteristics of dementia appear gradually; they may even temporarily disappear, only to recur to a greater degree. These characteristics include memory lapses and confusion, inability to carry on a conversation, and lack of interest in family life. They become over-dependent upon their caregivers and cannot see beyond their own problems.

They can't sleep, because they are agitated and restless; they often get out of bed and pace through the night. They express hopelessness of the present and the future. They don't trust anyone, especially those who care for them.

The dearest person can become a hateful wretch. Such a behavior reversal is hard on family members. Quite often, those nearest the patient forget that it isn't the patient but the disease that lashes out at them.

The Stranger I Call Grandma is a tool to provide both children and adults a better understanding of dementia, while helping them through the trauma of their situation.